I Brush My Teeth

Me Cepillo los Dientes

Written and Illustrated by McMillen Health
Texto e ilustraciones de McMillen Health

Translation by Darcy Lugo
Traducción de Darcy Lugo

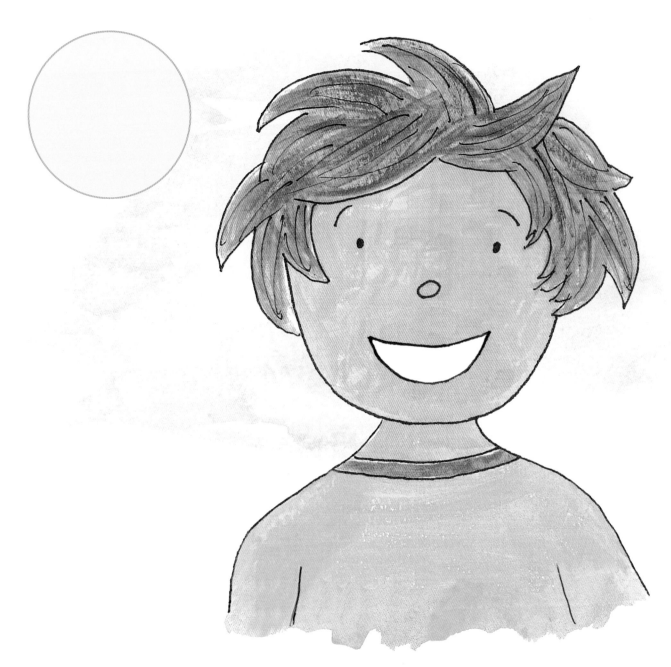

I brush my teeth in the morning.

Me cepillo los dientes en la mañana.

1.

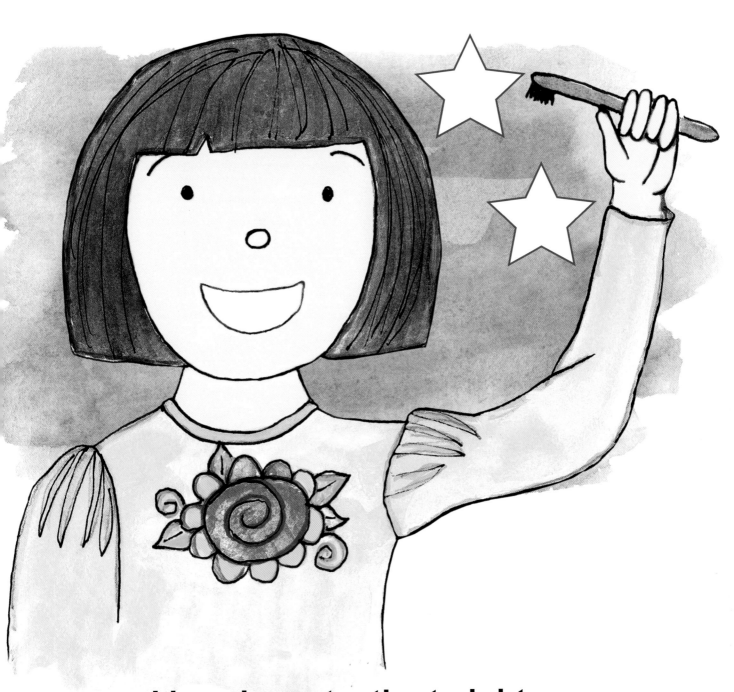

I brush my teeth at night.
Me cepillo los dientes en la noche.

2.

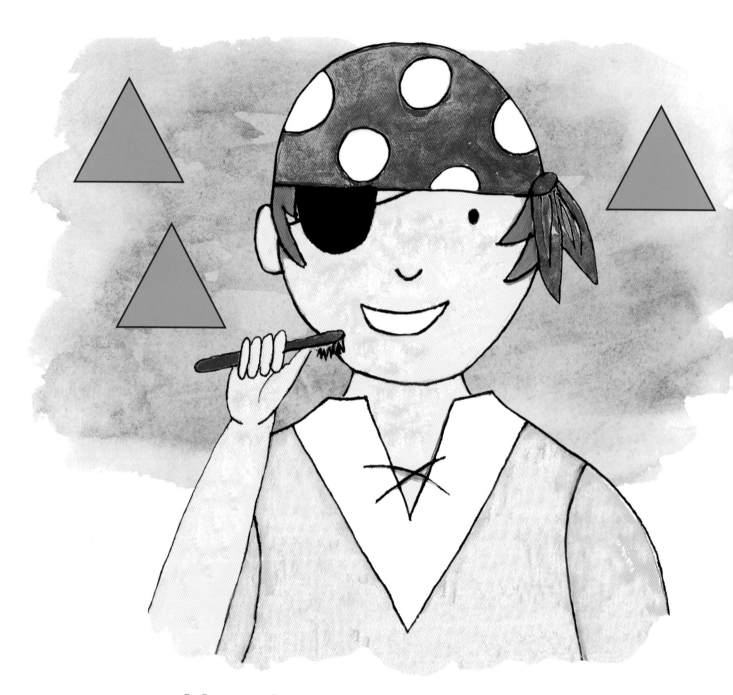

I brush my teeth on the left.

3. *Me cepillo los dientes de la izquierda.*

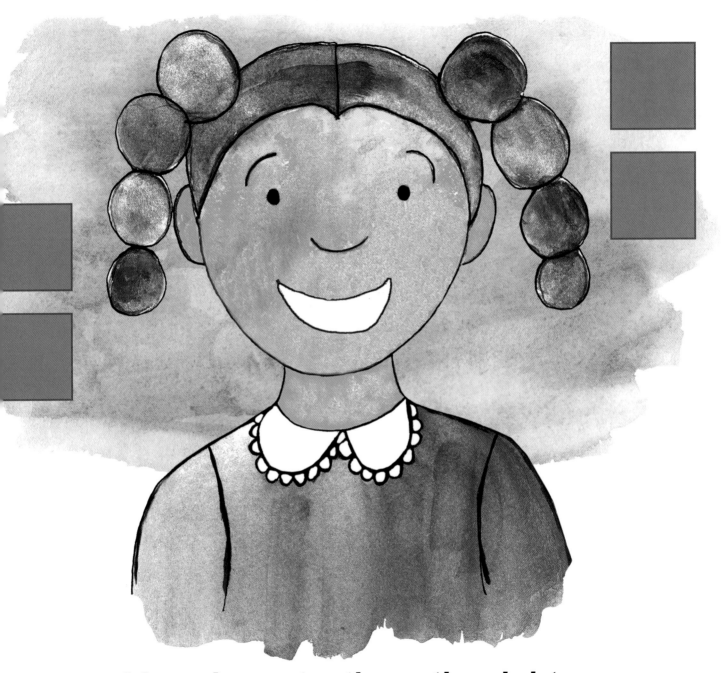

I brush my teeth on the right.
Me cepillo los dientes de la derecha.

4.

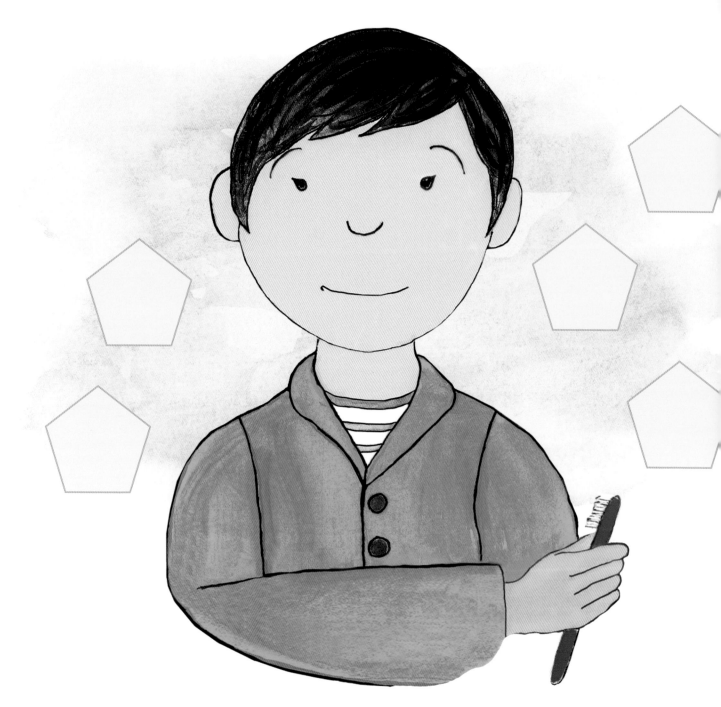

I brush my teeth on the bottom.
Me cepillo los dientes de abajo.

5.

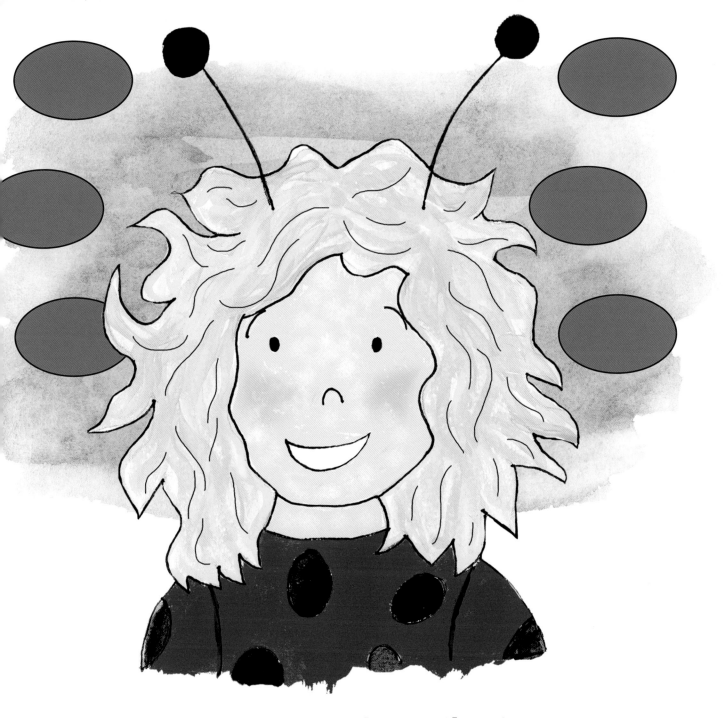

I brush my teeth on the top.
Me cepillo los dientes de arriba.

6.

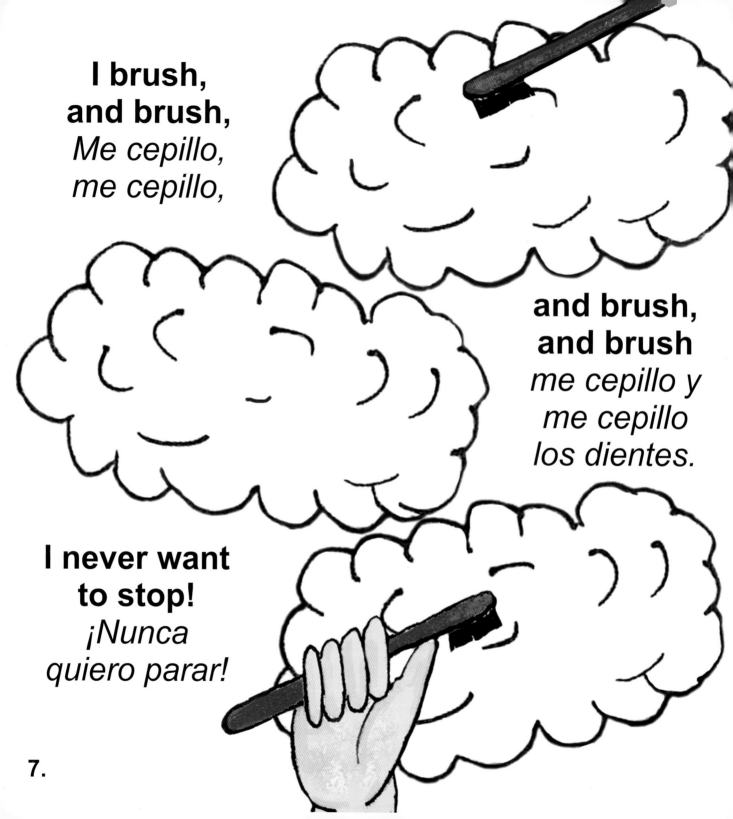

**I brush,
and brush,**
*Me cepillo,
me cepillo,*

**and brush,
and brush**
*me cepillo y
me cepillo
los dientes.*

**I never want
to stop!**
*¡Nunca
quiero parar!*

7.

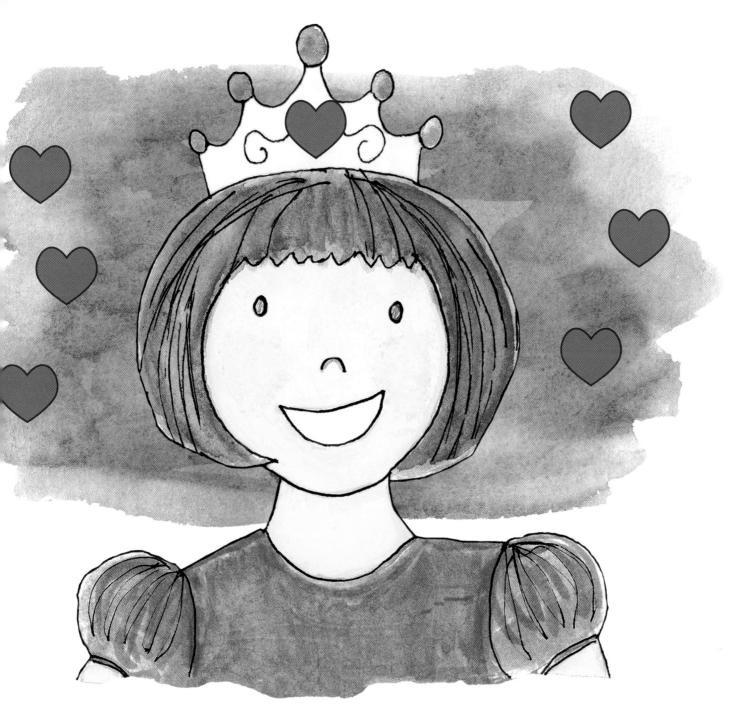

My smile is clean and healthy.
Mi sonrisa es limpia y sana.

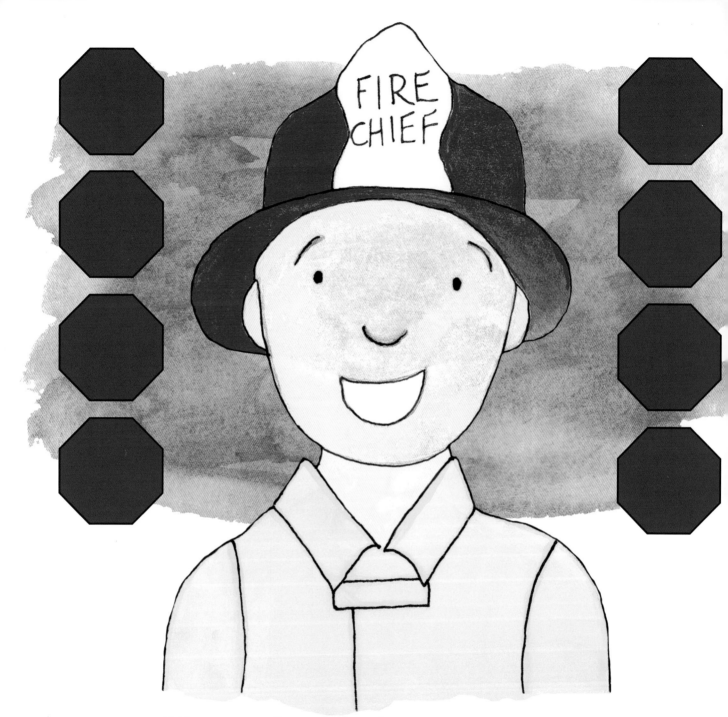

My teeth are shiny and bright.
Mis dientes son brillantes y luminosos.

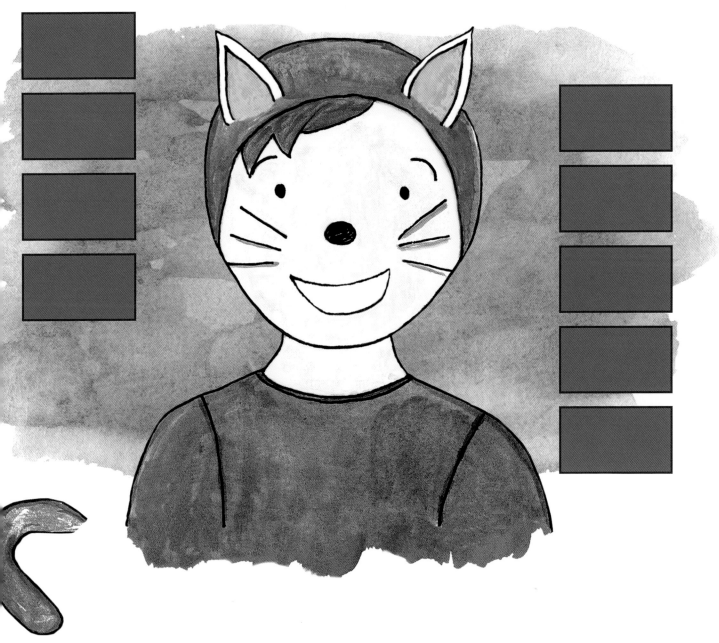

I brush, and brush, and brush, and brush.
*Me cepillo, me cepillo,
me cepillo y me cepillo los dientes.*

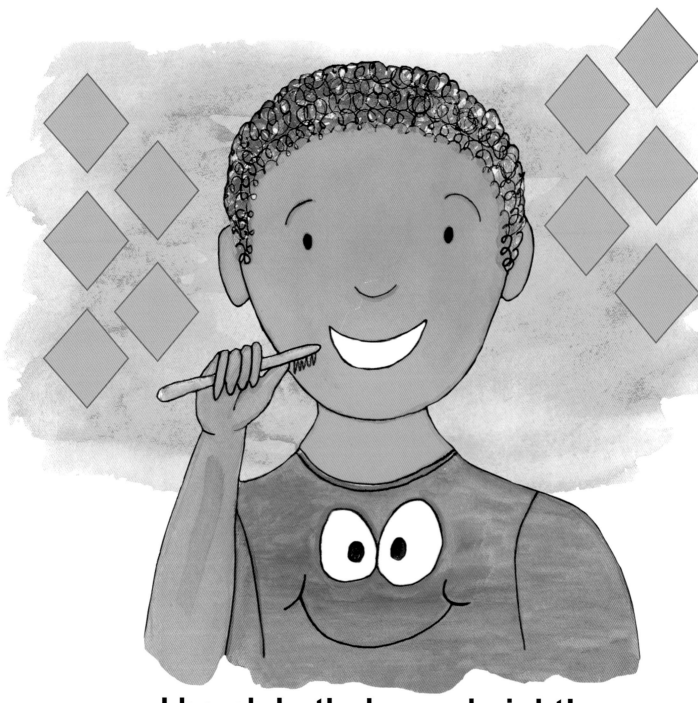

I brush both day and night!
¡Me cepillo los dientes día y noche!

PARENT RESOURCES
RECURSOS PARA PADRES

To help your child read this book, ask questions as you read. On every page, ask your child to tell you the color of the page. Have them name the shape and count the shapes.

Para ayudar a su hijo a leer este libro, hágale preguntas a medida que lee. En cada página, pregúntele el color de la página, la figura y a contar las formas.

On page 1, with the stars, ask your child to name other things they do before bed.

En la primera página, pregúntele otras cosas que hacer en la mañana, tal como vestirse o comer el desayuno.

On the pages where the children are wearing costumes, ask your child to name the costume. Ask them why they think the child is wearing a costume.

En las páginas con los niños de disfraz, pregúntele a nombrar el disfraz y por qué cree que usa el disfraz.

Ask your child what things they can do to keep their teeth healthy. Have them name some healthy foods they can eat. Talk about their favorite healthy foods.

Pregunte a su hijo qué cosas pueden hacer parar tener los dientes sanos. Pueden nombrar unas comidas sanas y hablar de sus comidas favoritas.

12.

On page 6, with the girl dressed as a lady bug, ask your child to point to the top of the page. Ask them what is at the top of their body (their head or hair).

En la página con la niña vestida como una mariquita, pregúntele a tocar la parte de arriba del libro. Pregúntele a nombrar las partes del cuerpo que están de arriba (cabello, cabeza).

On page 5, with the boy in a green sweater, ask your child to point to the bottom of the book. Ask them what is on the bottom of their body (their feet or shoes).

En la página con el niño en un suéter verde, pregúntele a tocar la parte de abajo del libro. Pregúntele a nombrar las partes del cuerpo que están de abajo (pies, tobillos).

Ask your child to name some things that hurt our teeth (like eating candy or drinking sugary drinks, like soda pop).

Pregúntele a nombrar unas comidas que dañan los dientes (azúcar, los refrescos, dulces).

When the book is finished ask your child to name their favorite picture. Ask them why it is their favorite.

Cuando terminan el libro, pregúntele su foto favorita y a explicar por qué es su favorita.

HAPPY READING!
¡FELIZ LECTURA!

Count the number of shapes:

Ayúdenles a sus hijos a contar las figuras:

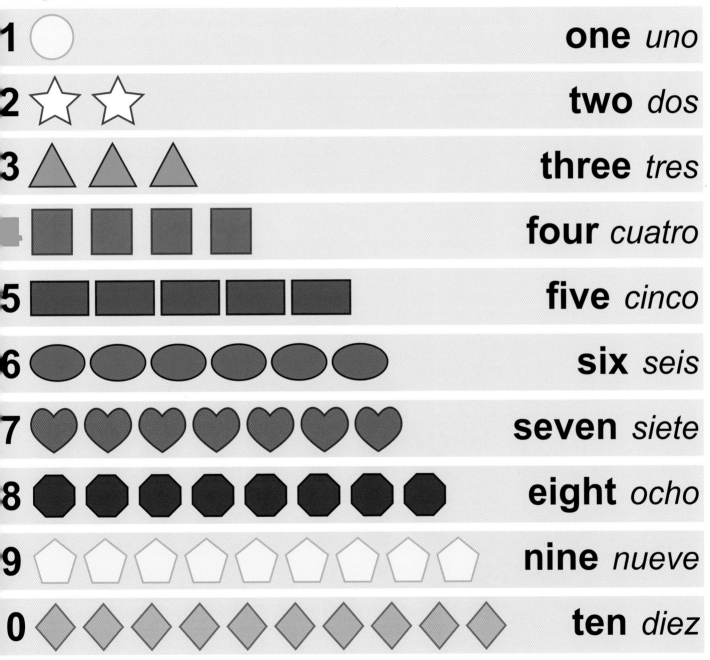

1 **one** *uno*

2 **two** *dos*

3 **three** *tres*

4 **four** *cuatro*

5 **five** *cinco*

6 **six** *seis*

7 **seven** *siete*

8 **eight** *ocho*

9 **nine** *nueve*

0 **ten** *diez*

Name the color:

Pregúntenles su color:

blue azul	**yellow** amarillo	**red** rojo
orange anaranjado	**pink** rosa	**brown** marrón
green verde	**white** blanco	**purple** púrpura